Memoirs of the

Pandemic

ISBN 978-1-71683-116-4
PRINTED IN THE UNITED STATES OF AMERICA

TABLE OF CONTENTS

* * * * *

PROLOGUE
Margo Nauert

On May 20th, 2020, the state of Illinois issued a stay-at-home order and closed all schools for a three-week period that ultimately resulted in the rest of the school year being taught at home via technology such as Zoom – a platform that was unknown to the general public prior to then. Words such as "unprecedented," "social distancing," "the new normal," and "flattening the curve," became commonplace. Toilet paper was a hot commodity, and it became clear that the pandemic that was working its way through the rest of the world had finally dug its claws into the United States. We could no longer ignore COVID-19. We could no longer compare it to the yearly flu. Infected or not, COVID-19 had an impact on everyone. Family members that I used to hug can now only be seen from six feet away. I worry incessantly for my elderly parents and my sister who works on the frontline.

Anyone can search the Internet to uncover the facts about COVID-19, but this book gives the feelings behind the facts. Like I stated, the virus affects everyone – young and old, and the students whose lives have been turned upside down, need an opportunity to share their voice. This is a compilation of journals, poetry, and photography from 6th grade gifted students. It is both heartfelt and inspiring. Today may be filled with anxiety, sadness, and tears, but tomorrow will come, and we will once again rise up having learned from the atrocities of today. So, take a minute and embrace these the words of our youth. According to Walt Disney, "Our greatest natural resource is the minds of our children." Take a step inside and look around.

~Margo Nauert

July, 2020

Journal Entry
Sophia Atanassov

Hi … I don't really know if anyone is ever going to read this, but I just have to get my thoughts out. Hopefully it will relieve some of the sadness. I am 12, and my name is Sophia. Just about a month ago, right before quarantine started, I was living my best life. On Thursday March 19th, 2020, I was at my last swim practice training for the relay at State. It was my first year in a USA Swim Team, and I couldn't believe I was even going. It usually takes people years to qualify for State. I heard that day at swim practice State had been canceled … well not cancelled, but the pool decided they were shutting down, so they had to find a new pool for us to swim in for State. Before they could even look for options, self-quarantine was issued. I remember that was also our last day of school.

Something weird was going on. They told at the end of the day at school over the speakers to bring our instruments home for the weekend. They never remind us, ever. I knew from that instant that we probably weren't coming back to school, but I just hoped we would. I never ever imagined how far this could come. I thought about one of my last memories there. I was on the bus, and the eighth graders and I were talking about it. One of them said that the band teacher hinted that school would be cancelled. Then another said there would be at least 2 people tested for coronavirus. My legs started to go numb, right as the bus started driving away to our houses. I didn't even look back. That is the first time I named it. My legs feel numb right now. Lots of people made jokes at school, but no one does that anymore.

My mom got an email saying school would be cancelled for 3 weeks. The first week they didn't have anything planned, so the teachers just gave us links we could go to. It was optional, and there was no schoolwork. The second week was when they started giving us assignments, and we have gotten one from every subject. The third was spring break. That Monday the 23rd of March, they let us go get our MacBooks, but I had already taken mine home. I went anyway because I wanted to get my schoolbooks. In case I needed anything. They didn't let me in at first, but then I said I had a book from the Carol Stream Public Library, and that's when they caved in. As our school officer led me to our room, as I walked through that gloomy hall, I saw all of the desks pulled out, and it smelled like disinfectant all over. I took my books, went out to my dad's car, wiped them at home, and laid on my bed for just a little while.

Then it kept getting worse and worse, we have the most cases in the world, over 450,000 and I don't want to look at the deaths, but I do know that more than half are recovered, and more people should know that. I miss everything, and I never realized how much you really appreciate things, until they are taken away from you. I have had a harder time with school every day, and I usually finish very late. I cannot get out that much and I feel sick. I need to get a fresh breath of air tomorrow, or I might just get emotionally sick. My head hurts. I thought that talking about things could let some stuff go, but it's hard. I'm tearing up, because nothing is certain right now. Maybe life might not ever be normal again, or maybe I might not make it. I might not be able to bake the cake on Friday. I am terrified, because deep inside I know that this pandemic has taken something away from my heart and from my soul that I can never take back. Sorry I need a little break. I cannot see the keys; they are blurry from my tears.

My dad has someone tested positive in his work facility, and he has to go to work every day. Let me just make one thing clear, I am really broken inside, and it really hurts. I am also in one of the better situations. I haven't lost a loved one yet, and I don't plan on losing one. My situation is nothing compared to the front-line workers, or the people that are hurting inside, or the people that are sick. This is nothing compared to everything else. And we will get through, one way or another, because we will learn to create a better future. We will fight through, to show that we can, and we will. We may lose many but save many more.

I know you may be reading this years from now, some of you might not remember anything about this time. Others of you might not even be born yet. But this is my story to share how it is bad, but everyday something good can happen. I try to get through one day at a time. I am speaking for every person out there, that is fighting for their life. We cannot see success without failure, we cannot rise without falling first, we might have made mistakes, but we have to remember this could have been worse. This virus will make us stronger, but we have to believe. And you will achieve in the end. No matter if this is months, days, or years from now. We will get through. The world will get through. Not without sacrifice, but without hesitation. I speak my word, for all of you that simply cannot, we will win. No pain No gain. And for the others that didn't experience it the way we did, just remember to live life the fullest.

I am going to be writing every day, and I have jars that I will fill as I write about a dream I have every day, a jar that I will write about something that was taken away, and a jar where I will write about something I can do during quarantine like bake a cake. I hope one day, that all three will be empty that I will get everything back, and that I will dream every dream I have. So just remember, don't waste your time with games, and movies, spend it with your family while you have them there. Go and travel the world. Achieve your dreams for the ones that cannot.

From me to you,

Sophia Atanassov

Journal Entry
Lauren K.

Wow, 10 weeks of being stuck at home (I think). Not too long ago I had a discussion with my sister saying that we have been doing online learning for 10 weeks, but she said that we had been doing it for 9 weeks. She was right because we had one week off of online learning for spring break. Yay, a trip to my living room! But it has felt like an eternity since I have been in school hanging out with my friends. I just wish I could go back for even just a day so I could see everyone. But I can't. Will we even start next school year in school? Or will we be stuck doing our first few weeks of schoolwork online? Right now, there are no questions that can be answered correctly. Nobody knows what there is still to come.

Well, I do have one exciting part about my life right now. I get to start up softball soon! I have a tournament up in Wisconsin in a few weeks, and I am super excited. Then, at the end of July I am going to Kentucky for nationals. The only bad part about all this is that a few rules have been changed. We still play the game the same way, but nobody can go into the dugouts and parents will either have to watch from the outfield or sit in their cars for the whole game. There are still a few other smaller rules that have been changed, but in general it all means to stay away from others and social distance yourself. I'm just excited that I even get to play.

I just hope that everything gets back to the way it was before COVID-19 really sprang into action. I know that online learning is about to end, and that summer vacation is coming up, so I will get to take lots of trips to my living room, basement, and kitchen. Yay me!

-Lauren

JOURNAL ENTRY
Savan Patel

Life has been weird these past couple of months. All of our lives have been different - from school all the way to just going outside. Going outside is kind of like a life or death situation because of Coronavirus. School has been really different because we have to do remote learning where we do our homework online. We can't see our friends except on zoom calls.

Another really big issue that applies for most people is boredom. Boredom is taking over most people because we have nothing to do except stay inside all day. My schedule has been basically the same every day, and I want it to change. People who do sports have to stop playing and they probably can't even practice. Also, people who actually have the virus are having a very hard time fighting it. Lastly, there are the healthcare workers who are on the frontline fighting the virus and risking their lives. Life right now is definitely not the same.

~Savan

JOURNAL ENTRY
Sophia Atanassov

What is the situation we are living in really feeling like? It is very different for everyone, but I think one thing we have in common is the unnatural feel of it. I wake up 2 hours later than I would on a regular day, and I have this feeling like I don't have to do anything because you have nothing to look forward to. My mom is working non-stop since she has to deal with all the network issues they have, my dad still goes to work, and I just have to get my schoolwork done to watch my little brother. I miss looking forward to school, and I miss going to swim. I am afraid that if I go back to school my grades might go down, or if I go back to swim, I won't be able to get best times and qualify for State. The rest of my family lives in another country. I cannot see them, I cannot go back there this summer, and the uncertainty of this situation scares me the most.

I don't know when this will end, when quarantine will end, when will we get a normal life again. Will life ever go back to normal? I guess if you are reading this it might have, or maybe it is different than before. I don't know, the teachers don't know, and the world doesn't either. The cases keep going up and down and up and down, without really giving a clear signal of decline. I wish I knew what will happen, because I have an unknown future ahead of me. Everyone does, but in this situation, you don't know if you will get the opportunities you wished for. I wanted to travel the world and explore the Great Barrier Reef before it is all lost due to bleaching. Will I ever be able to even do one dream that I have set in mind? We will have to see. The only real certainty is that we really don't know a good amount about anything that is going on, and I hope that people will learn from this, because no one really deserves living like this.

~Sophia Atanassov

Journal Entry
K. Edwards

Life has been very stressful during the pandemic. I don't really have anything important to be stressed about; there are some people in much more harmful or bad situations, and I can't even imagine how they're feeling because all I've got is some schoolwork and me not getting it done, that is stressing me out. I try to get some of my work done, but then I forget about others and I just end up watching YouTube. That is all I'm stressed about.

I heard that the government is helping people pay for their taxes and living expenses for people without jobs. I think that the way the government is getting all the money to help people is by printing it, and this is really going to devalue the economy because there's going to be more money existing, and so therefore money is going to be less valuable. Now things are going to be more expensive and people who aren't getting financial aid from the government will struggle. All their money is being devalued and they're going to have to start paying more and it's going to do some pretty bad things.

I'm just saying it's just been a really scary time for everybody, not just me. But I'm glad that my point of view is going to be somewhere where you can help people in the future. I really wish that this never had to happen. I wish we could take it back, but we can't, and it is happening, so I'm glad that I get to be here and witness it with everybody else. It's a horrible thing to have to live through and to see how it's affecting other people but it's also going to be a major historical event, and I guess I'm kind of glad to be a part of the people telling the story and showing people how things can be affected and that someday somebody might learn from our experiences.

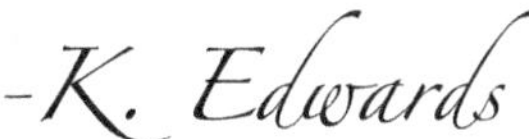

Journal Entry
Emmaline Kovich

I don't really know where to start, but I guess I'll begin with our last week before we left. It started out just like any other week, but as it went on, it seemed like many of the teachers were getting prepared for school to be cancelled. I think it really started to sink in for everyone when they called us all down to get our band and orchestra instruments and bring them home over the weekend. We had Friday off that week, and so it was going to be a longer weekend, but they still have never made a big announcement like they did that day. We all kept asking the teachers if school was going to be cancelled, but none of them could give us an answer because they were just as uninformed as the rest of us. Most of the after-school activities were cancelled that day, so almost everyone was on the bus. The bus is always so fun and gets your mind off of things, so on the bus that day I wasn't really worried about anything because we were all just having a good time. Little did we know that that was going to be our last bus ride together of the school year.

That Friday both my sisters still had school since they are in high school and my dad was at work, so it was just my mom and me at home. In Governor Pritzker's press conference that day, he was going to announce if the schools were closing or not. I really wanted school to be closed because I was ready for the year to end. Obviously, he did announce that all Illinois schools were going to be closed until the end of the month. At first, I was happy, but then I realized how much I missed going to school, even though I was so ready for it to end.

The first week that we had e-learning we didn't have any work assigned because our school district wasn't prepared to begin distance learning. The week after that we had actual e-learning where each teacher would assign work for their subject. At the start most of our work was easy and was to just pass the time and get your mind off of the craziness going on in the world. Once we got farther into e-learning and were informed that school was cancelled for the rest of the year, the work started to get more challenging and even more educational.

After two weeks of being out of school, we had spring break. My family and I had so many plans for spring break, and it was disappointing that we couldn't do any of them. I think that it also brought me to an even deeper realization of how much this really is affecting everything. Even though we had already been quarantined for two weeks, doing e-learning and still having somewhat of a sense of normalness made things not as real. But when we were on spring break, all we could do was find something to do in our house or backyard and that was it.

My oldest sister, Amalia, is a senior in high school, and the rest of her senior year was completely ruined. I feel really bad for her and everyone else in her situation because there are so many big events that happen the last few months of your senior year. My other sister, Lily, is a sophomore in high school and she is in driver's education this semester. Since she can't finish her drivers ed. course we don't know when she will be able to get her driver's license. I'm grateful that I don't have any major milestones that are supposed to happen this year for me, and I feel bad for anyone that is missing out on something that they have been looking forward to for a long time.

I think that one of the worst things about this whole situation is that you are scared of people. It is so weird to be afraid of interacting with a person. Some people in my family are at higher risk, so we have also had to be more careful which makes me even more scared to interact with other people. I'm more worried for not only me to get it, but to spread it to the people that are at high risk and could have a harder time recovering.

During this crazy time, I think that many people have been stressing and worrying about so many things. I know that I have been very concerned and anxious about the pandemic. A few weeks into quarantine I had a panic attack because everything was just so overwhelming and a lot to take in. There have been many nights where I can't fall asleep because my mind won't slow down and just wanders and thinks.

Even though quarantine has been hard, and I have known a few people that have gotten COVID-19, I am grateful for the situation that my family is in. There are many people that can't feed their families right now or are losing businesses that they have worked hard for because they cannot afford it anymore. Even though I have known a few people who have gotten the virus, they have all recovered and ended up ok. It may seem hard right now, but I know that we will get through this and everything will be okay again.

~ *Emmaline*

Journal Entry
Zack T.

At first, people were skeptical. "You're overreacting." We all joked and talked about it. No one thought that the world would ever have a full blackout. It was unexpected. We can't leave the house?! Some people followed. Some didn't. We grew as a society, with positivity, with negativity. This all started by bat testing in Wuhan, China. China was never the best country. Was there fighting? Yes. Racism and people going crazy. Not just in America, but also in China. "Chinese virus." "#BlackChina" "Africans being evicted from their homes." The impact was somewhat terrifying. People have to stay inside or go outside, worrying about dying.

The president isn't the best during this time. He is the ruler of one of the most powerful nations. He was never...smart or the best. He's one person but truly not good enough.

My life? We now have online school. We wake up, work, and go back to sleep. School was the one thing all of us are used to. It's a routine. Losing it is like moving homes. Some people hate it. They don't work anymore. Some people miss it. It can be a distraction from home. Domestic abuse, partner abuse. They can't escape it now. The small things are now an issue. Getting a haircut, cooking, cleaning, refurbishing, it's all we can do now. We're forced to work as a society without being together as a society. Home is school. Home is life.

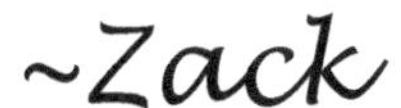

Journal Entry
Lauren K.

What is happening? What is the government hiding from the world? Why only negative in the media? So many unanswered questions. I want to know what is to come. I only know now and the past. COVID-19 is spreading fast from state to state, from city to city, from home to home. It's everywhere.

I am stuck in my house but go out on the weekends to take a bike ride. I have to avoid people on the sidewalks and ride my bike in the grass because I don't think people truly understand the social distancing rules, stay 6 feet away from others.

Because I am stuck in my house, I cannot go to school which means I'm doing online learning. Kids say that they don't like school or don't want to go, but now that we are in this position, kids actually want to go back and be in school again. I want to go back soooo badly. Also, my softball season was put on hold because of this. I was looking forward to a tournament inside the Chicago Bandits' dome. Now, I can't even go to practice. It all feels **terrible**. I just wish this would all end so everyone can get back to their normal lives, but that's not happening. Coronavirus has had such a great impact on the world that it's going to be a while.

-Lauren

Journal Entry
K. Edwards

Thursday, April 30th
Week 5 of Quarantine

I'm so bored. I'm starting to get into a routine, but the days feel so short. My days are around 12 hours and they feel like 5. If my homework wasn't constantly reminding me, I would forget what day it was. I am so out of the loop of life and I feel like I am not moving forward in life or accomplishing anything.

-K. Edwards

One week until we are done with online school
Still in Quarantine

I'm excited to have all day with my family in summer, but I am also sad because of the Coronavirus. I will not have a lot to do. My brothers and I are digging a giant hole in the backyard, so that will occupy me for some time, and I also have the book I'm reading so I guess I'm glad, but I will miss my classmates and teacher and I'm sad I will not be able to end the year with them.

K. Edwards

PHOTO JOURNAL
Sophia Atanassov

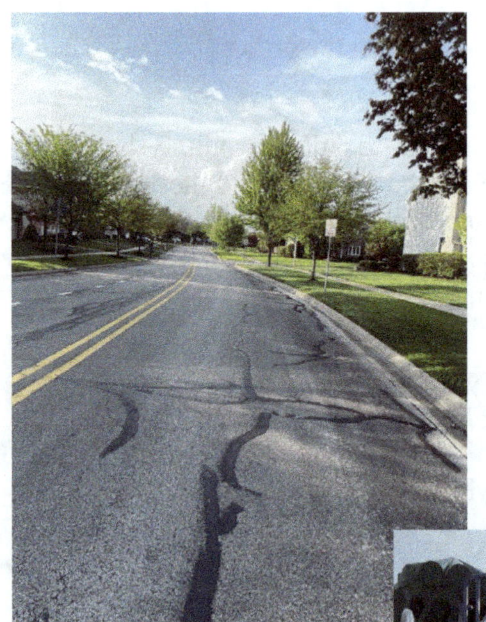

Empty streets

&

Closed parks

Closed

Schools

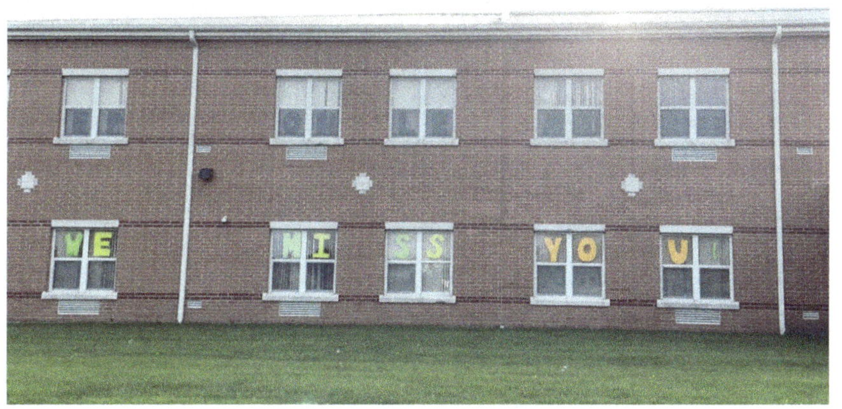

A Metaphor
Lauren K.

Right now, we are like an erupting volcano. Our emotions pouring out of us like lava flowing down a mountain. Happiness has been taken over by sadness, calmness has been taken over by the worries of the world, and all these negatives have multiplied. It feels like our world is crashing down on us. But we can get back up and rebuild our lives like they were before. Rome was not built in a day, and neither will our future, but we can still do it.

LIFE RIGHT NOW
Zack T.

Life is an apocalypse
Life is full of fights
Life has more deaths
Life has the happy
Life brings the bad
Life is how you choose it
      Happy?
          Sad?
Whichever are you?
How will you make your life?
Full of fighting?
Full of helping?

Life has society
Society shows two
      Terrible?
          Joy?
The terrible give misery
The joy gives positivity
Will you do either?
Will you help society?
Is there anything you can do?
      No?
          Yes?
Are you useless?
What can you do?
Think of your answers
Think of the people
Think of others
Think of their life
      Will you?

Life made the apocalypse.
Society changed the apocalypse.
Are you making a change?
Are you stopping the change?

Will anyone stop this apocalypse?

LOVE STRONG REALITY
Lauren K.

L oving
O thers,
V alue
E veryone

S tay in
T here,
R ise up
O nly,
N ever
G ive up

R eal and
E verywhere,
A reas
L iving
I nfected lives
T rue? . . .
Y es

POETRY OF THE PANDEMIC
John L.

A Collection of Couplets

My "at home" haircut looks bad
And now I am sad.

Toilet paper everywhere,
But there's never any to share!

Mask, mask, here and there
They protect us from stuff in the air.

There's a meat shortage
So I'll go eat some porridge.

Don't know when quarantine is gonna end,
Might be 2021 or the weekend.

Ah, staying home;
It's very monotone.

A Collection of Triplets

I need to get healthy,
So that I don't get a big belly
While sitting in front of the telly.

Package;
It's very neat
And also sometimes a cool treat.

Going to the grocery store,
Needed lots of butter.
Wanted to make lots of cakes for my mother.

A Collection of Haikus

Now it's end of May.
Quarantine started in March.
When's it going to end?

Quarantine is weird.
But Zoom calls are kinda fun.
Now I have homework.

A Collection of Quatrains

I woke up at seven
Or so I thought
When I checked the time
It was actually eleven!

If I had a dollar
For every time someone went out
I would then say 'holla!
'Cause I get lots of clout.

Going outside,
It's very nice;
But flying worldwide,
And you'll pay the price.

I really want to go to the park,
But all of them are closed.
I guess I'll just go to my backyard with wood bark
And lots of stuff that's decomposed.

I got me a workout
That's really cool
But then I get tired
And I sleep and drool.

Hoarding, Hoarding,
Why does it exist
It sounds a bit boring
And I don't get the gist

Woot woot!
Got 15 hundred dollars
Woot woot!
Gonna go holla!

9:00 every day,
Have to go learn.
After that I can go play,
And tomorrow I'll return.

Been doing lots of stuff
That I was supposed to do before
It's sometimes really tough
And I always get more.

Poems are weird;
Words that are cool
There're kinda engineered
And some are about drool.

Staying at home;
Feeling like cabin fever.
Can't go roam;
Unless I was a beaver.

Zoom, zoom,
Better get going
'Cause of my meeting
And I am also not slowing

Cough, Cough,
Sniffle, Sniffle,
Do I have it?
No, it's just allergies!

A Limerick

There was once a guy in his home
Who lived in the city of Rome
When he went outside
Everyone would go hide
'Cause he wasn't supposed to go roam

A Cinquain

'Rona
Sickness around
Cough it and you are sick
Caused whole world to be in lockdown
Virus

A Definition

How's it like living in this pandemic?
A bit boring.
I love sleeping in.
FIELD TRIP TO THE BEDROOM!
I have eaten so much.
Why isn't my Internet working?
I do not know if it's Monday, Thursday, or June.
Yikes!

Coronavirus went around everywhere,
From Wuhan, China to London, U.K,
Shutting down the world and causing a scare,
Causing the world to turn down and be gray.
Started in China, Wuhan to be quick
Before the day 2020 began.
Small pneumonia cases with a kick
Started out small but then death, hitting man.
But the world went "Stop It!" and tried to fight
Quarantine, social distancing galore.
People tried to help with all of their might
But we need to drop cases down to the floor.
When this is over, I'd like to say
Thanks to everyone who helped it to sway.

MEMOIRS OF A PANDEMIC
Lauren K.

Negative thoughts start pounding through my veins
Families give a loved one a last kiss
Lots doing this... feeling the biggest pains
Scared kids asking, "Can you tuck me in Sis?"

All of this stays forever and ever
Coronavirus running through the air
Will it stop? Will it go away? NEVER
Whoever gets it, is it really fair?

I hope, and I'm sure I speak for all,
That no one in my family gets it
I don't want to get that terrible call
If it happened, I'd throw a crying fit

When this is over and about to end
I hope all ill patients are on the mend

PHOTO JOURNAL
Lauren K.

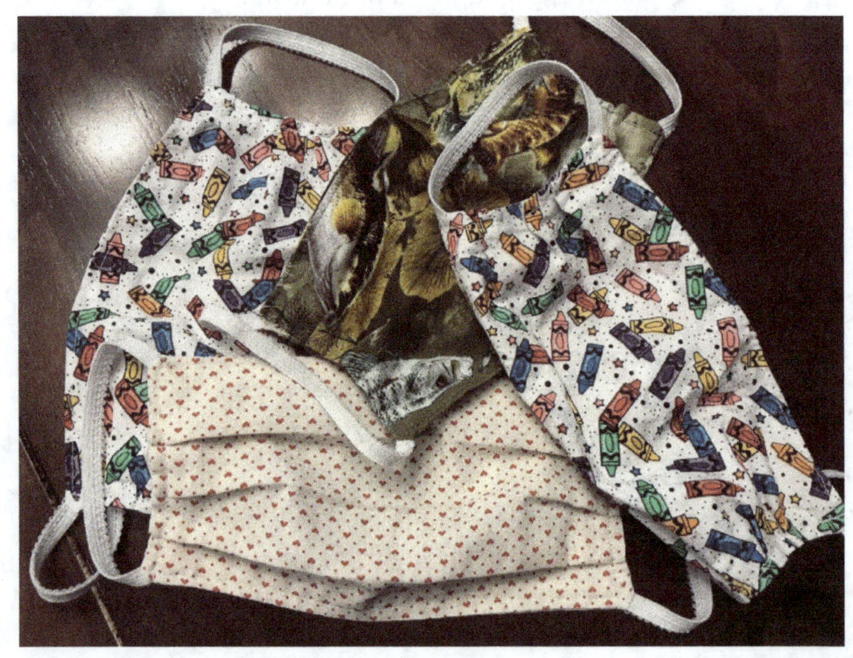

The Latest in Fashion

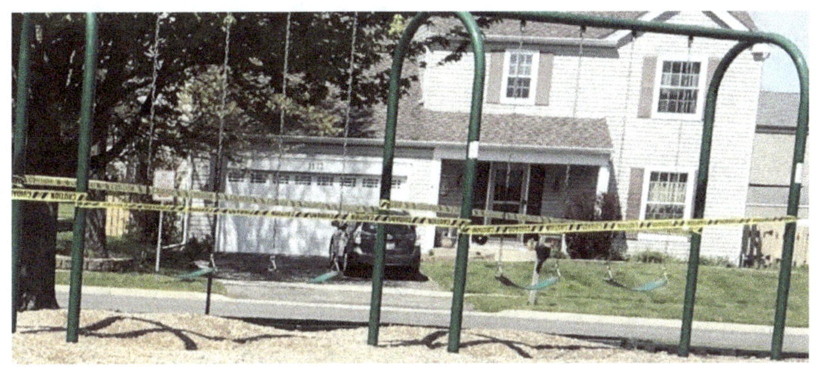

Nowhere

   to play

     &

No one to see

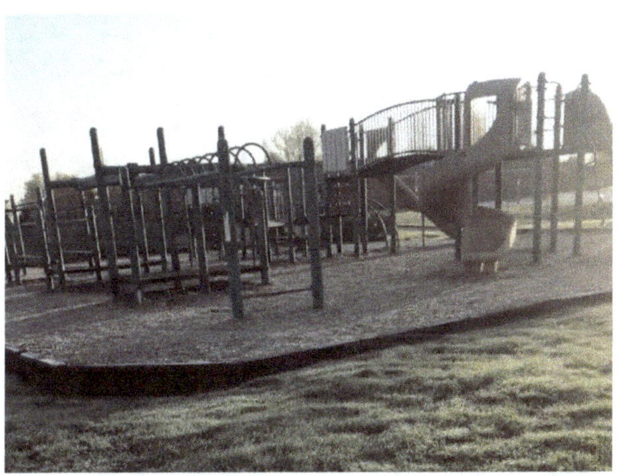

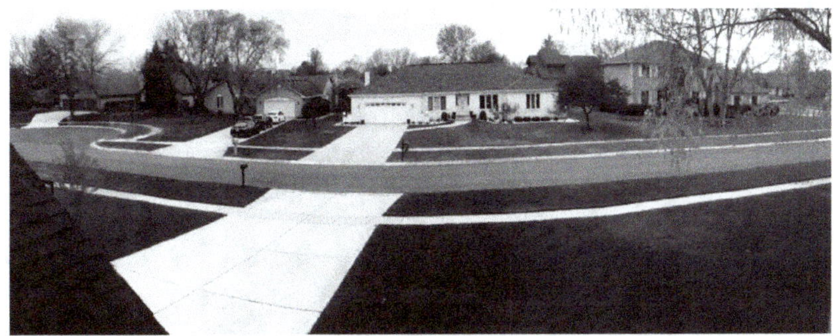

A Tribute to Surviving The Pandemic
6th Grade Gifted Class

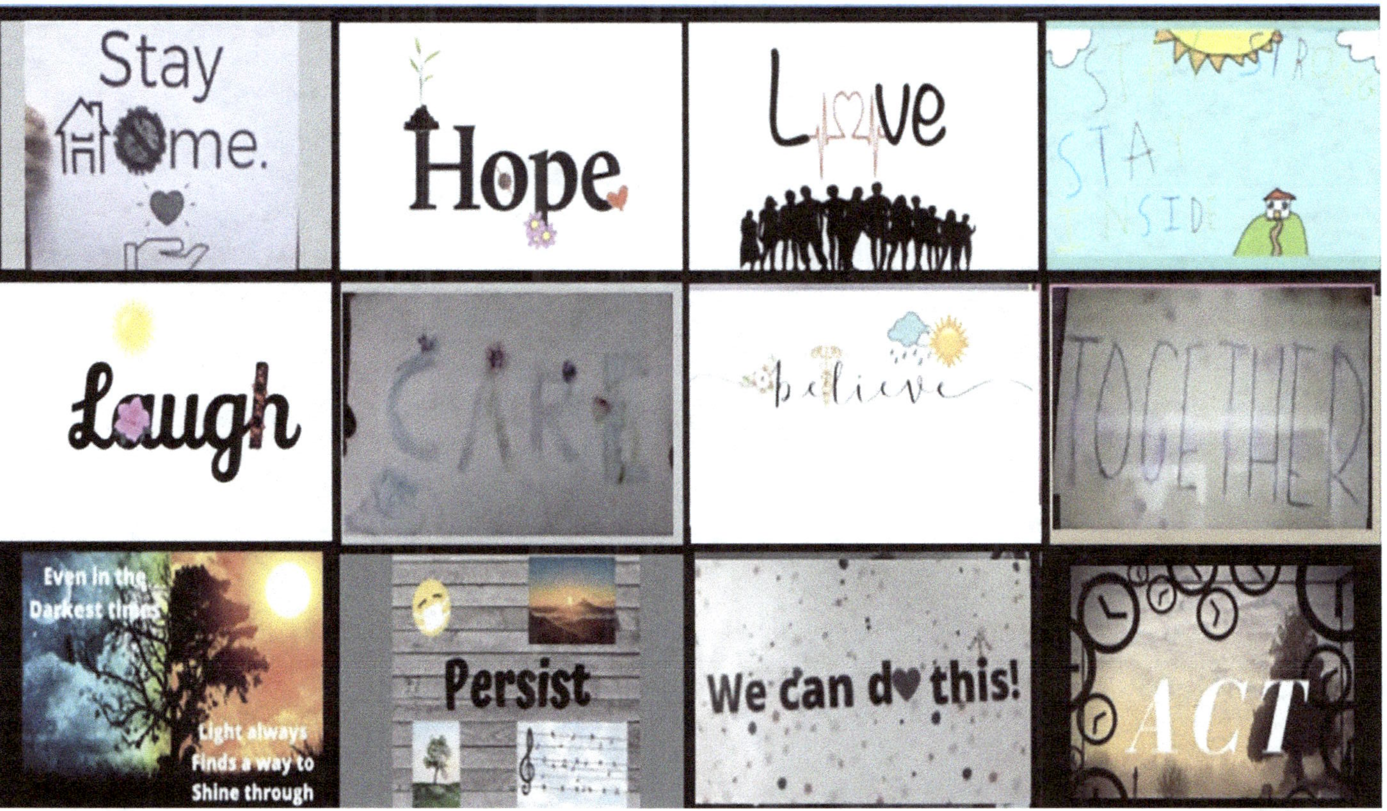

Stay Home.
Hope
L♥ve
Stay Strong Stay Inside
Laugh
CARE
believe
TOGETHER
Even in the Darkest times
Light always Finds a way to Shine through
Persist
We can do this!
ACT